Table of Contents

Comprehensive Study on the Causes and Treatment of Childhood Asthma

Exploring the Causes of
Childhood Asthma

1. Introduction to Childhood Asthma

It is now generating a significant amount of research in regards to the origin of asthma because of the increasing number of children who develop asthma and other related allergies, in particular, in Western civilizations. Asthma is a chronic inflammatory disorder that particularly affects the bronchial tubes and is characterized by recurrent and inevitably reversible airway limitations. Asthma affects 5-10 percent of people worldwide. In addition, social, economic, genetic, and environmental factors are thought to contribute to the etiology of asthma. The role of inflammation in early life in the original asthma has intensified efforts to identify measures to prevent the occurrence of the disease development while the immune system is malleable. As a result, a better understanding of the causes of allergies is needed in Western society.

Asthma is a complex and multifaceted condition that affects the bronchial tubes. It, in particular, makes breathing a difficult task and is also fast-spreading. It has been estimated that about 500 children in every 10,000 in high-income countries are susceptible to being affected by this condition. Many of these children go on to develop severe chronic asthma after the age of three years. Acceptance of the theory that the disease is caused by a multiple set of factors has been widely embraced. These factors encompass both the fetus' genetic and environmental condition and the child during early years. Exposures to oxidative stress factors during fetal and early childhood while the immune and lung tissues are developing are considered the most essential. The innate and Th2 responses are increased due to exposure, increasing the likelihood of developing asthma. In contrast, the size of the bronchial tubes is also reduced.

Childhood asthma is a significant disease process that is increasing in prevalence. Prevalence rates of asthma among U.S. children almost doubled from 3.5 percent in 1980 to 6.2 percent in 1994. The data also reveal the following information about prevalence rates by various factors. For U.S. children, prevalence rates of asthma were reported higher at traffic-dense locations compared to locations with low traffic. In the International Study of Asthma and Allergies in Childhood (ISAAC) multicenter study, the mean prevalence of ever having diagnosed asthma was 13.8 percent, with national rates closer to 20 percent. The mean prevalence of lifetime wheezing was 27.6 percent, and the mean prevalence of at least one symptom (wheeze, rhinitis, or eczema) was 26.0 percent. Asthma was more common among boys than girls, except for in the Caribbean and South and Central America.

Childhood asthma is a disease process that is characterized by lower airway inflammation, hyperreactivity, and obstruction. The primary symptom of asthma is a non-productive cough. Other symptoms include wheezing, barrel chest, and clubbing of the fingers. Additionally, the disease process has a greatly negative impact on the quality of life of the patient. Public health nurses must educate their pediatric patients and their families about the pathophysiology, causes of symptoms, and measures that can be taken to control the disease process and therefore improve quality of life.

2. Genetic Factors

A genome scan for asthma was conducted using a whole genome panel of microsatellite markers to genotype 487 British sibling pairs. Strong evidence for linkage to asthma was seen in a region on chromosome 7p. This study suggests the presence of a gene involved in the etiology of asthma within a region on chromosome 7p containing the protocadherin beta gene cluster, providing further support for the suggestion that beta-catenin-dependent WNT signaling pathways make a contribution to the genetic risk of asthma. Genetic factors contribute significantly to the development of asthma. Specific inherited factors that have been very strongly linked to susceptibility to asthma in multiple studies include single-gene definable diseases and specific polymorphisms, such as 21-hydroxylase mutations in congenital adrenal hyperplasia. Hereditary factors inherited include atopy, total IgE, and bronchial hyperreactivity. Asthma prevalence is greater in those children whose fathers have asthma rather than not have asthma. Grandparental smoking increases the prevalence of unsensitized asthma. Total IgE and bronchial hyperreactivity have been shown to be inherited. Hereditary factors contribute to 40-42% of the variability of asthma in children. Twin studies have shown allergic sensitization to be highly heritable, varying from 70-83% for food allergies or inhalant allergies. The inheritance of asthma is variable, where 36-79% of childhood asthma cases were inherited, while 45-67% of asthma cases appear sporadically. The rate of inheritance of asthma may also vary depending on the severity of the disease, with up to 76% of moderate to severe childhood asthma inherited. Since HRV infections have been associated with asthma outbreaks, one may assume that genetic factors that predispose to HRV infections may also predispose to the development of asthma.

Childhood asthma is a condition common in modern western societies and its incidence is increasing. The fundamental causes are still not clear and likely prospects include genetic susceptibility or exposure to environmental insults in early life. Evidence of heritability comes from clear familial patterns and migration studies. Although an increasing number of chromosomal regions involved in asthma and asthma-related traits have been described, the identification of the causative genes has proved more difficult.

2.1. Family History

• Parental history of asthma • Maternal age below twenty • Cigarette smoking by parents (they allow kids to smoke) • Parental cigarette smoking before birth of a baby (in-utero exposure) • Decreased outdoor air quality (life phase pollutants) • Having trouble with drinking water • Possible exposure during the early years of life (3-4 years) to environmental tobacco smoke (ETS) The history of asthma suggests that a kid could inherit asthma, however a family history of asthma may be more, partially since it prefers or favors exposure to the family allergens, partially as parents with asthma may raise their child in an atmosphere with better recognition and perception of the disease which leads to a faster diagnosis of asthma in a kid.

Childhood asthma is a heterogeneous disorder. There is no clear general cause of the condition. Instead, several contributors promote the likelihood of getting the disease. Childhood asthma is indeed partly inherited or familial. It is essential to keep in mind, however, that there should not be any single cause of asthma. Hundreds of genes can interact with a variety of potential environmental parameters to induce asthma in a single child. Subsequently, asthma is likely inherited through a complex but often determined genetic mode known as polygenic inheritance in which dominant and recessive genes are present and establish the degree of risk for each predisposed child. An atopic child (i.e. allergic to aeroallergens or foods) with familial asthma has a significantly increased risk. Family tone of atopy such as eczema and allergic rhinitis also raises the likelihood of getting asthma. Factors contributing to the cause of asthma include all of the following or variable types of connected data.

2.2. Genetic Mutations

We also identified genetic mutations causing defects in other pathways that interfere with the normal development of our immune system in children and increase the risk of them developing severe asthma. So, in one of our recent studies, we screened coding and gene regulatory regions for both known common variants and rare coding variants linked to a panel of genes that encode molecules associated with asthma. A total of 10 novel variants were identified in seven genes, namely PGAP3, FSD2, HAVCR2, TSLP, VDR, IL33, and KLRB1. Thus, the much granularity and data analysis can provide an indication of different asthma causative mechanisms in children. Some of the different variant genes were found to encode functions in both the structural and immunological pathways and are discussed in the final paper. Only little overlap was found for common or rare variants between mild and severe asthma genes, indicating separate genetic pathways at the level of variant risk for these three asthma characteristics.

Genetic mutations can predispose children to developing asthma. These genetic alterations may not be the sole cause of asthma, but they may contribute to how early someone can get childhood asthma, how severe asthma can be, and how kids respond to the treatments. Genetic mutations that are found to increase the risk of childhood asthma include coding variants in the growth receptors, interleukin 33 (IL-33), and Vitamin D receptor. These receptors are responsible for growing and differentiating T helper cells that regulate the immune system in our body. The growth of T helper lymphocytes is known to be at lower levels in kids developing severe asthma as adults, as proved in one of our previous studies, which only highlighted growth receptor variants.

3. Environmental Factors

Qualification of environmental factors considered for inclusion in this review was based on the evidence regarding the potential for contamination of the PAHS profile by additives, such as creosote. Airway function during the early life stages of asthma development is generally underdeveloped and smaller; thus, airway hyperreactivity due to exposure to pollution persists for a longer duration among asthmatic children. The nature and intensity of interactions parents and caregivers have with children, as well as the types of play and physical activities children may engage in during different seasons or times of day, are likely to depend on individual family customs, during clinic visits or conversations with the caregivers, parents, children, or family. In particular, indoor formaldehyde exposure from personal home products. The presence of negative effect mediators and/or confounders such as the child's sex, parental smoking, or socioeconomic status is also possible when conducting longitudinal cohort studies, through assessment of possible subpopulations with a higher risk of cytokine coding exposure.

Experts postulate that environmental influences, including exposure to multiple pollutants and allergens, significantly contribute to childhood asthma development. Indeed, findings from experimental studies have shown that varied allergen and non-allergen exposures during the prenatal period may influence fetal immune programming and, consequently, increase the risk of asthma with attacks or exacerbations early in childhood, although subsequent exposures can modify the severity. The factors of exposure, type of study participants, and study settings may also have a significant impact on these findings.

3.1. Indoor Allergens

In infants, several studies have demonstrated that living in a home with indoor allergens is a significant risk factor for the later development of asthma. During the development of the immune system, exposure to these allergens can occur, resulting in skin tests that are IgE positive in 69 to 100% of the allergic children exposed to these indoor allergens. These allergens also remit and produce spontaneous skin tests. It is in these allergic children that chronic inflammation and smaller respiratory tubes occur, with pulmonary function tests indicating reduced mid-expiratory flow, and consequently greater airway resistance. Several larger studies show these indoor antigens do not have any influence on the health of the general population, but do have a strong effect on those allergic to these childhood allergens. Each of these can lead to allergic symptoms proceeding to chronic inflammation (asthma allergies and eosinophilic infiltration of the bronchi), and bronchial hyperreactivity (BHR), the components of asthma.

3. Indoors. What is it in the indoor environment that affects childhood asthma? Several studies support that allergens fill that category. 3.1. Indoor allergens - Indoor triggers can produce an immune response leading to asthma symptoms. There are several asthma-causing factors in the indoor environment including house-dust mites, furred animals, cockroaches, mold, and others. Additionally, cockroach stool and saliva that are not antigens can also lead to an allergic asthma response.

Outdoor Allergens: Scientific literature has demonstrated that outdoor plant and insect allergens and irritants affect the incidence and severity of asthma among children. For example, one striking American study provides clear evidence for the growing seriousness of allergic diseases in children. Data from the National Health Interview Survey revealed that the number of children under age 18 who suffered from pollen allergies grew from 6.5 percent in 1997 to 9 percent in 2002, representing a 38.5 percent increase in five mere years. The medical installment estimated that fully two million children have pollen allergies and more than four million kids under the age of 18 have suffered from asthma symptoms in a given year. The most common outdoor allergens are pollen and tiny particles from cucumber, bamboos, and grasses. Because these allergens are common in the environment and can travel for miles, pollen is harder to avoid than virtually any other allergen.

Asthma is a chronic condition that affects the airways, causing them to swell and produce excess mucus. Asthma makes airways more sensitive, which can lead to symptoms such as chest tightening, shortness of breath, cough, and wheeze. Environmental pollutants, such as outdoor allergens and chemicals, can irritate children who have asthma. Researchers are examining the relationship between these environmental factors and asthma in the hope of preventing the illness from developing and improving asthma management. In this section, we will focus on the three primary outdoor elements that can contribute to asthma development and exacerbation in children. These include outdoor allergens, which we will discuss in this part. The two remaining environmental pollutants will be reviewed briefly in other sections. They include outdoor air pollution and tobacco smoke.

4. Exposure to Tobacco Smoke

In children exposed to maternal smoking, airway inflammation already begins in the prenatal period, worsening during and after birth. The inflammation involves the upregulation of the mRNA for many inflammatory markers, upgrading inflammation. Maternal smoking during pregnancy was also associated with increased wheezing. Children exposed to antenatal maternal smoking, who are allergic and exposed to secondhand smoke (SHS) at home, might be the subgroup that presented with the highest levels of fractional exhaled nitric oxide and peak exhalation flows (PEF).

During pregnancy, smoking interferes with the normal development of the lungs, leading to a reduction in alveolar number and size of alveoli, with long-term sequelae. The persistence of small and large airway obstruction and increased hyperresponsiveness in early adulthood may exacerbate the deleterious effects on the lung of any noxious agent exposure, concomitantly enhancing the development of a persistent asthmatic aeropathological profile.

Exposure to tobacco smoke is one of the most important factors in the development of childhood asthma. Several metabolic and hormonal changes have been demonstrated to be potentially related to the chronic or even occasional maternal smoking during pregnancy. These changes can have consequences in the respiratory health of the children, leading to asthmatic symptoms. It seems that the presence of the father's tobacco smoking does not have an additional impact on lung function when the mothers smoke.

During gestation, pregnant women transfer maternal nutrients and chemicals to the developing brain, liver, and circulation of the fetus. Cell types responsible for immune responses, regulation, memory, and youth are at differing points of development during the nine months of gestation. Subsequent studies have since determined that exposure to tobacco smoke in utero detrimentally impacts lung structure and function into adolescence and possibly adult life. Consequently, prenatal smoke exposure has been associated with an increased risk of developing asthma in childhood. Indeed, the school-aged children and adolescents of mothers who smoked during pregnancy are more likely to be diagnosed with an asthma-associated condition compared to the children of non-smoking mothers. Collectively, the altered lung structure, abnormal immune responses, and increased risks of lower respiratory tract infections during childhood culminate to amplify the risk of a child developing childhood idiopathic asthma.

Asthma is a common chronic health condition in children, which can manifest as a coupled set of symptoms comprising chronic airway inflammation, bronchial hyper-responsiveness, and recurrent episodes of reversible airway obstruction. It is widely established that maternal smoking during pregnancy is linked to the occurrence of childhood asthma. Consequently, numerous international bodies advocate for informing expectant mothers about the consequences of smoking and recommending or arranging some type of help or support to quit. In the past, the educational system and public health services have instead employed stigma and neglect to shape the behaviors of new mothers and traditional 'responsibilisation' approaches have not worked to improve the respiratory and overall health of our youngest generation.

4.2. Secondhand Smoke Exposure in Childhood

Secondhand smoke alterations can occur as early as before birth. Mothers who smoke while pregnant may slow their children's growth of airways, which results in increased airway resistance and risk for asthma development in their children. Newborns exposed to tobacco smoke since birth have higher serum IgE levels than their unexposed counterparts. By the age of three months, these children have respiratory symptoms of cough and wheezing. Babies living with smoking parents have four times as many respiratory problems as babies living with non-smoking parents. Nicotine and cotinine, the major metabolite of nicotine, which are the two most toxic and kept for the longest amount of time in the body, cause increased airway responsiveness and airway inflammation. Chronic exposure to secondhand smoke among children and adolescents is associated with an increased prevalence of respiratory conditions, particularly asthma and wheezing. Thirdhand smoke can affect the functionalities of human primary nasal epithelial cells similarly to secondhand smoke.

Accumulating evidence from various studies in recent years has revealed that secondhand smoke exposure in childhood is one of the leading risk factors for asthma. Secondhand smoke, also known as environmental tobacco smoke, contains over 4000 chemicals, of which at least 250 are known to be harmful and more than 50 are known to cause cancer. This section explores the effects of passive smoking on childhood respiratory systems, leading to asthma development.

5. Respiratory Infections

Other respiratory pathogens may interact with allergy to exacerbate asthma symptoms. Mouse data indicate that virus and allergen co-exposure acts synergistically, so that immune mediators induced in asthmatic lungs following virus infection amplify the allergic tissue response; in humans, such interaction between infection and allergen has been investigated, supports the role of immune mediators in perpetuating the occurrence of asthma. High levels of house dust mite allergen in the bedclothes of young children with an untreated wheeze were previously shown to predispose to new wheezing exacerbations, and more recently to result in new asthma or asthma symptoms. RSV bronchiolitis in infancy can completely block subsequent sensitization to the allergen cat within a medium-sized population, but at age 13 is associated with an at CT diagnosis of asthma or emphysema only among pre-adolescent children previously sensitized to cat - a finding of a dominant sensitization source tied to major domestic allergen exposure resulting in enlarged airways.

Respiratory infections. Viral infections are widely recognized as significant triggers for asthma exacerbations. Reports over the last two decades have confirmed that preschool wheeze often occurs post rhinovirus infection, the most common viral trigger of asthma exacerbations. Rhinovirus infections early in life have been shown to disrupt lung growth, possibly resulting in children with reduced lung function who are more likely to develop asthma than to recover. Other suggested viral causes of childhood asthma include other respiratory viruses which cause either reduced lung function, wheeze and bronchiolitis or viral bronchiolitis, and viral factors such as the presence and amount of interferon, which can either diminish viral replication or augment inflammation underlying later asthma. It has been suggested that such viral infections could themselves induce allergic sensitization and thus be directly associated with allergen-induced asthma exacerbations.

5.1. Viral Infections

Induction of asthma symptoms Activated and memory/effector Th2 cells with eosinophilia form the main adaptive immune response in the asthmatic airway, both as a cause and effect of increased airflow obstruction. This prototype of cellular outwebbing in the airway of asthmatics is driven by acute viral infections and toxin-induced systemic immune administration and regulation. Asthma is a chronic inflammatory lung disease initiated by genetic and environmental risk factors interacting in complex ways. Exacerbations are mainly of viral origin. Major questions are: (a) how do environmental factors lead to sensitization and regulation, (b) how do these regulations lead to exacerbations from time to time, and (c) how do the subsequent pathologic processes combined with co-morbidities advance to chronic symptoms? In bronchial biopsy and induced sputum of childhood asthma, allergen-induced combined signs of neutrophilia and eosinophilia and severity-positive Th1 immune response developed under negative CD28 regulation of T cells have been shown. In childhood asthma, airway hyper-reactivity has been connected with fewer CD25+CD4+ regulatory T cells.

Causative viruses of asthma in childhood Several viruses can be involved in the pathogenesis of childhood asthma. The primary responsible is the human rhinovirus, followed by respiratory syncytial virus and adenovirus. Immunoglobulin-E-mediated allergy is acquired via the skin mainly very early in life. Later, children encounter a series of respiratory virus-induced exacerbations of their disease at the peak in years 3 and 4, and the cumulative aspect of infections contributes to the later onset of 'apparently new' disease. In summation, viral infections are an essential key to several aspects of childhood asthma, including the following: (a) they are responsible for governing the precise location of the most frequent asthma symptoms along the bronchial tree, (b) they lead to inflammation that affects women more than men, (c) they play a mediating role in the association of lower respiratory tract infections and asthma, (d) they are the major precursor of chronic wheezing whenever it occurs.

6. Diet and Nutrition

Food allergies have long been identified as a specific risk factor for asthma in children. Often, children avoid activities that promote asthma, except for when such activities are done in clinical settings. For this reason, the adult population is often studied. Research that has explored the relationship between diet and asthma prevalence amongst adults has shown that excessive levels of various dietary components, such as protein, carbohydrates, and caloric (energy) intake in general can have an impact on one's health and response to illnesses. One commonly studied food-related factor that has been related to asthma – specifically, asthma training – is obesity. Current clinical guidelines have not included diet or obesity in the treatment or management of asthma. This is because, although obesity is associated with the development of asthma among adults, it is not the only potential explanation for the development of asthma. Moreover, obesity is not required for sedentary lifestyles! In the future, the influence of obesity and other food-related factors – such as antibiotic use – should be explored in the context of pediatric asthma.

Childhood asthma is a complex condition that results from the interaction of many different factors, some of which are unique to individuals and some that are more widespread in children generally. Despite the fact that we cannot identify or predict the factors that will lead to an asthma diagnosis in any specific child, researchers have worked to discover the populations that are at a higher risk for asthma than others, and one of the risk factors that has more abundant research behind it is dietary and nutritional factors that impact asthma development.

6.1. Obesity

Asthma is a typical chronic disease in childhood, affecting approximately 14 million kids worldwide. According to the World Health Organization, the problem's magnitude is so great that it merits major consideration. Asthma attacks among children are also rising, particularly in countries like Canada, the United Kingdom, and sometimes the United States. Moreover, gender variations are reported in some of these nations; for example, more boys are diagnosed with asthma than girls in the United States. An improvement in health, nutrition and hygiene facilities may be attributed to the worldwide decrease in asthma attacks. Despite these initiatives, there has been no change in childhood asthma rates, let alone a decline. The prevalence of obesity and being overweight has increased in children over 20 years, with children having the greatest obesity and being overweight rates. Furthermore, because of diet, comprehension of the incidence of children with asthma and obesity is essential.

The incidence of obesity in males and females under the age of 20 continues to be high. Excessive weight has more negative effects than just excess pounds; it may also raise the risk of developing other health problems, such as hypertension, atherosclerosis, non-alcoholic fatty liver, metabolic syndrome, type 2 diabetes, and numerous chronic diseases. According to some research, asthma is more common among obese children than among children of regular weight because of a diet higher in n-2 polyunsaturated fatty acids (PUFA). PUFA are abundant in vegetable oils such as soy, maize, sunflower seed, cottonseed, and sesame, as well as in nuts and seeds. Some of the dietitian's roles are to assist in the development of educational programs and materials to inform the general public about the role of dietary fiber in maintaining healthy body weight, for the early identification of persons at risk for health problems, and to educate them about the state of being overweight and the negative outcomes of obesity.

7. Allergic Sensitization

Researchers said the findings are significant because the Caribbean region has one of the highest documented rates of wheezing illnesses in the world, an unexpected adverse effect of increased urbanization, industrialization, and large-scale urban renewal of cities in tropical and subtropical regions. The incidence of asthma jumps from one in 20 children in the U.S. to about one in 20 children to as many as one in five children in some island nations in the Caribbean, where the burden of the disease and its contributing risk factors are not fully characterized. Asthma is responsible for many hospitalizations, missed school days, and a decreased quality of life. Fortifying the link between early allergen exposure and new development of childhood asthma in Jamaica will greatly inform the planning, prevention, and treatment of pediatric asthma in the region, they said.

Allergen sensitization significantly raised the odds of developing asthma if co-occurring with another underlying health problem, researchers found. Allergen sensitization, when combined with virus-induced wheeze in the first year of life, at two years of age in the Caribbean region carried a 10-fold increased odds of developing asthma by age 5, researchers said. "Early allergen exposure increases the risk of childhood allergic diseases," Courtenay Moore, a doctor of medicine, pediatric resident, and clinical researcher at the University of East Anglia, Norwich, U.K., said. "This study classically demonstrates the negative effect of allergen exposure in developing respiratory health in Jamaican infants and young children."

Children with allergic sensitization to Blomia tropicalis, a common house dust mite found in the Caribbean, at three years of age were four times more likely to have developed asthma by age 5 than children without, according to University of East Anglia researchers in Jamaica. Sensitization to either cockroach or mold allergen at age three was associated with a 2.5-fold higher risk of new-onset asthma by age 5, they reported at the virtual American Academy of Allergy, Asthma & Immunology Annual Meeting.

7.1. Early Allergen Exposure

Exposure to allergens early in life might contribute to the development of asthma in two ways. First, exposure to multiple allergens at an early age might increase the risk of allergic sensitization and subsequent asthma early in life. Secondly, sensitization to multiple allergens might be more strongly related to more severe asthma, whereas the presence of multiple allergen sensitization later in life might not substantively affect asthma severity since the asthma might be controlled by other mechanisms. Infants who are hypersensitive to allergens are those who develop the most severe asthma. Early allergen sensitization and early-late cumulative multi-allergen sensitization have been associated with increased severity of asthma. Hyperresponsiveness to inhaled corticosteroid medications and severe allergic sensitization further increase the severity of asthma. Severe, poorly controlled asthma in childhood usually persists until adulthood. Early wheezing is usually triggered by infections and not by allergies. However, infections also play a role in the development of wheezing.

Allergens are the primary causes of asthma in children. Children who are sensitized and display symptoms when exposed to allergens at an early age are far more likely to develop chronic childhood asthma. Environmental allergens may trigger an asthma attack. Pollens, fungal spores, domestic mites, cockroaches, pet dander, and secondary tobacco smoke are some of the environmental allergens that trigger asthma. Therefore, early identification of sensitization to environmental allergens is essential. It has been suggested that children possibly begin immune gp24 response to allergens during the first year of life. Allergen-specific IgE and associated increased levels of pro-inflammatory cytokines like IL-4 and IL-13 are more commonly seen in children less than 3 years with allergies. Early sensitization to allergen in very young children in the first few years of life results in non-atopic asthma in childhood.

8. Stress and Psychological Factors

Claesson and colleagues performed a longitudinal study to assess the risk for asthma of 5557 children with stress-related disorders. Children with similar diseases, including separation anxiety, reactions to severe traumatic events, and social relationship problems, showed a higher risk for an adverse outcome compared with children with stress but did not have any stress-related disorders. Maternal stress is a strong factor related to difficult-to-control asthma. Different asthma reviews and studies have shown that stressful events in families can exacerbate asthma in children. Maternal stress is one of the primary factors for reduced illness perception in asthma management, which worsens the disease. This indicates that maternal psychological factors and symptoms must be evaluated, should be included among the adverse outcomes of the disease, and must be further examined in pediatric research.

Several psychosocial factors, such as mental stress and psychological disorders, have been examined as potential contributors to both asthma pathogenesis and its adverse outcomes, including exaggeration of symptoms and a decrease in daily life activities. It is not yet fully understood how stress can directly induce airway inflammation or affect asthma. Notably, several studies have reported a significant association between stress-induced decrease in lung function and a significant induction of airway responsiveness with allergens in sensitive children. Stress is a common trigger for asthma symptoms in many children. Parental stress early in life is a risk factor for the development of asthma in childhood in extremely preterm infants, particularly among those who are colonized with S. aureus, and can also predict the onset of wheezing and/or a diagnosis of asthma during childhood.

8.1. Parental Stress

In this survey, 460 parents and caregivers of 401 children aged 0 to 19 years with asthma and 459 parents and caregivers of 353 children aged 5 to 19 years without asthma from 10 schools in Andalucía, in Southern Spain. Data on asthma status were obtained via the International Study of Asthma and Allergies in Childhood (ISAAC) written questionnaire designed for children aged 6 to 7 years (5 to 7: parental complete version) and adolescents aged 13 to 14 (11 to 14: adolescent complete version), both of which included a module about psychological topics. Parental HRQOL was assessed by using the Spanish version of the Short-Form-12 Health Survey (SF-12) and the Spanish version of the 12-Item General Health Questionnaire (GHQ-12), on the psychological well-being, and parents and children completed the Asthma Pediatric Quality of Life Questionnaire (PAQLQ). In multiple conditional logistic regression analyses, we found that carer identity, the perception of the child and the child's life event were all independent risk factors for developing asthma. The parental and children HRQOL was worse when parents and caregivers reported that their children had more severe asthma. The HRQOL of parents and children was worse when both parents and carers and children reported that children had higher levels of negative emotional responses. Although the possibility of reverse causality cannot be discounted on the basis of this survey, the mental well-being and HRQOL of individuals in families caring for children with asthma and diverse degrees of severity were more impaired.

Parental stress could result in psychophysiological changes and poor mental well-being, which have been found to be associated with the development of asthma in children. Female caregivers and parents have been studied more often than male caregivers and parents have, which may limit the research to female caregivers and parents up to now. We used a family-based methodology to examine the association between parental psychological status and the occurrence of childhood asthma, particularly how parental stress and parenting stress and child life event might have an impact on children and how, in turn, children with asthma influenced their parents' mental well-being and HRQOL.

9. Hygiene Hypothesis

The hygiene areas, such as handwashing and cleaning, can negatively impact the development of the microbiome in infancy and the subsequent risk of developing atopy and/or asthma. Cuts in hygiene are needed to protect us from diarrhea, which is the most global killer of children and infants. It is more likely that poor lifestyle changes, poor diet, poor childhood-rated stress, antibiotic abuse, vitamin D deficiency, or an increase in Caesarean section rates can trigger our immune systems to respond inappropriately. Th1 responses are suppressed and become more allergic in the appropriate genetic predisposition. The hygiene hypothesis is the cornerstone of our knowledge of childhood asthma, and evidence supports it. But it is not a simple cause. Allergy and asthma are multifactorial. The hygiene hypothesis suggests a role of infections as a possible culprit. It is an area that requires more research. Test these ideas.

The hygiene hypothesis has been around for many years, and it is based on the finding that children who grow up on farms and have many siblings experience fewer allergies and asthma. The hygiene hypothesis is a statement that in children, Th2 responses to allergens are suppressed, and their immune systems are trained to express Th1 cell responses to possible pathogens. The microbiome develops appropriately, and the risk of asthma is reduced. This idea has grown into a book, demanding that exposure to early infections, farm animals, and a diversity of bacteria can protect children from developing atopic diseases or allergic responses.

9.1. Microbiome Development

Higher normalized abundance of Streptococcus in the nasopharyngeal microbiome of infants and toddlers at 2-3 years of age is associated with increased asthma risk later in childhood. At 6-12 years of age, linear correlations between asthma risk and normalized abundance of Streptococcus in question of an association with Streptococcus SPF were no longer present. Instead, the children with the second-highest normalized abundance of overnight Streptococcus SPF had the lowest asthma risk. In conclusion, children with an excessive microbiome reaction have a lower asthma risk, and feverish disease indicates a reaction strong enough to affect the microbiome. Thus, the microbiome may serve as a disorder marker of hypersensitivity in all cases. A possible future mark of disease can also be the sum of different bacteria with the strongest impact on the bronchial lymphocyte cytokines. If this is the case, then the chemistry behind the illness can be understood by understanding the effect of the bacteria on lymphocytes.

The hygiene hypothesis for asthma is closely linked to the development of the microbiome. Children living in rural areas with animals, day-care attendance, elder siblings, and other factors leading to crowdedness experience an earlier maturation of the microbiome with a richer flora than children living under more hygienic conditions. This has led to the idea that a delayed maturation of the microbiome might be involved in the development of asthma. However, the relationship between microbial exposure in early life and the risk of asthma is complex, as asthma risk has been shown to be associated both with early day-care and pet keeping on the one hand and a delayed maturation of the microbiome on the other hand.

10. Conclusion and Future Directions

One of the few protective factors for childhood asthma that has received relatively consistent validation to date is growing up on a farm. This is likely to be achieved via a different route than that via which endotoxin leads to a reduced prevalence of atopy and atopic disease; however, the size of the effect of protection from asthma, compared with the reduced risk of atopy, is less well defined. Exposure to endotoxin in infancy has received attention elsewhere as a potential treatment after birth to reverse existing wheeze; potential causal pathways are outlined in figure 1. The evidence for area-level air pollution causing childhood asthma is clearest in the area of particulate pollutant effect, although it is not strong enough for it to have been considered a new cause by WHO/IUATLD in a review of available evidence conducted a decade ago. A number of other pollutants have also been considered as a cause of asthma syndrome but have received little investigation to date because of a lack of evidence.

Asthma is one of the most common chronic diseases in childhood and adolescence. Its high prevalence, particularly in developed countries, suggests a role for the environment (both in utero and after birth) in causing or promoting one or more of the likely causes of childhood asthma that have been discussed in this chapter. In particular, we have elaborated on the role of viral respiratory infections, endotoxin, vitamin D, and air pollution as potential causes of asthma, concentrating on plausible mechanisms and the most convincing resulting evidence. Although possible, the role of the fetal environment as a direct cause of asthma has received the least investigation to date. A clearer understanding of the effects of the environment on asthma causation would guide advice about measures that could reduce the current unpleasant levels of asthma morbidity in children.

Comprehensive Study on the Causes and Treatment of Childhood Asthma

1. Introduction to Childhood Asthma

Let us begin this comprehensive study with the definition, distribution, and symptoms of this squint-eyed and twisted disease in our precious children to define the subject in a scholarly manner towards its causative factors and the sequence of diagnosis and treatments with references. Childhood asthma is characterized by reversible airway obstruction and hyper-responsiveness of the airways. The reversible obstruction in the airways could be either complete or partial, and both lead to the reduction of airflow to the lungs. As it is reversible, so the complete treatment of asthma is a possibility. In the case of children, the symptoms of this disease vary in their ages. Some major symptoms have been observed in children having asthma. It has a high rate of morbidity and mortality in the pediatric age group. Many etiologies are involved in the pathophysiology of childhood asthma.

Asthma is a heterogeneous disease, usually characterized by chronic airway inflammation. It is defined by the history of respiratory symptoms such as wheeze, shortness of breath, chest tightness, and cough that vary over time and in intensity, together with variable expiratory airflow limitation. This common airway disease is the most common chronic disease in childhood, affecting 10-20% of all 6-7-year-old children of each population. There is a high rate of remission of asthma in children, but 3-10% of adults (depending in part on prevailing levels of risk factors such as obesity, smoking, infection, and pollution) are likely to have a combination of chronic cough, sputum production, and airway obstruction. Worldwide, regardless of the child's age, asthma is associated with significant morbidity, impaired physical activity level, altered emotional state, time off school, impact on the family; in some children, the disease can be life-threatening.

1.1. Definition and Prevalence

Asthma is defined as a condition of the respiratory system that can vary in severity from mild to severe, characterized by airway inflammation and increased airway reactivity to a variety of stimuli. The term childhood asthma refers specifically to the condition's attacks starting primarily during childhood. Prevalence of asthma has been increasing during the last few decades in affluent societies. In developed countries, as many as 20%-25% of children have been reported to have at least one asthmatic attack by the time they reach the teenage years. The urbanization process and environmental pollution notably are thought to be major contributors to this increased frequency. In developing countries, the prevalence varies from one country to another, and even in some affluent societies, the frequency is lower, ranging from about 5% to 12%. As a chronic inflammatory disease, childhood asthma is the most common chronic disease in childhood and is reported to have a considerable impact on children's daily life. It also has significant effects on families and incurs financial burdens related to medical service use and insurance costs as well as parental work loss. As asthma's symptoms are quite different in children compared to adults, the standard adult-based diagnosis of asthma is not applicable to children, especially those with recurrent wheezing or exaggerated coughing. Consequently, epidemiological studies become important in understanding the true burden of childhood asthma in effective healthcare planning and allocation of resources. Also, mothers and caregivers witnessing the ailment alone at home and noting relevant symptoms are also affected by the signs and symptoms children suffer, not the disease itself.

1.2. Impact on Children's Health

It is clear that the disease has various repercussions for the overall health of the developing child, including nutritional status and emotional distress. In some studies, asthma has been associated with a lower quality of life due to the many symptoms and fears it may manifest in the child and family. Asthma is relevant to the area of mental health in children because of the many complications in diagnosis, treatment, and parenting during attacks. The impact on the child is of great importance. The disease's physical impact on the child is very disturbing, including factors that can be monitored, such as lung disorder, which may indicate the development or severity of the disease. Identifying and understanding the health impacts, including the treatment of the disease, are basic steps to assess the significance of asthma and to improve the necessary attention and management. A better revision of control measures can be done based on correct data from a global to a local level. Open recommendations and attention to distinct impacts are necessary, while multidisciplinary research can be performed to present diagnostic and therapeutic tools in an integrated manner, using available evidence, to guide asthma care from birth. Therefore, the aim of this study was to explore the effects of asthma on the development of children based on available evidence. The focus is on sources of knowledge that are frequently and deeply investigated, referring to the most pertinent evidence, monitoring different procedures and progress in the work, and clarifying specific aspects that are often inconclusively explained among those involved in care and health activities.

Having an asthma attack can be a terrifying experience for the child, secondary to choking spells associated with difficulty breathing and lightheadedness. It is very common for parents or caregivers to have harmful thoughts, experience guilt, or face restrictions on activities, interests, and social isolation that children may encounter because of their condition. There is often a marked lack of support. These mental health disorders are not directly related to the severity of the condition, but rather to the concerns and worries of those who cannot do anything to help their children during acute attacks.

2. Causes of Childhood Asthma

Asthma is the most common chronic pulmonary disease in children. There is clear evidence that asthma results from complex interactions between genetic, environmental, and behavioral influences. Since these interactions start in early life, it is assumed that the origins of asthma are very often grounded in early life. This article attempts to disentangle the complexity of these different factors causing childhood asthma. By doing so, we aim to contribute to a better understanding of the different levels of underlying processes resulting in the development of asthma in children. And second, we argue that the identification of different causes and mechanisms might aid in the development of treatment and preventive strategies that better match the individual need of asthma patients. There is growing evidence that common triggers of asthma such as air pollution, allergens, or nutrition have different consequences for biological systems depending on the underlying (genetic) processes and the age at exposure. Information about lifetime health risks exists for populations in general, and many healthcare systems are organized on the basis of population health. It will take much more effort, but also offer the best opportunities for better treatment, to extend the knowledge base towards the individual child. Therefore, most of the results of this review are based on findings in the pediatric population (age range defined as 0–18 years). Asthma is a complex disease. As reviewed earlier, most pediatric cases of the disease are driven by a variety of exposures hastily following the first breaths, some of which will be health promoting, some will be health compromising, with the majority simply ineffectual. Each initiation of the asthma process, sometimes referred to as an insult of programmed events, has the potential to launch a program of development into childhood and beyond in which the child looks and feels well (clinically well) while showing early signs of abnormal physiological, somatic, metabolic or psychological function. Those with such early pathways of development for-provoked asthma may progress in later life to possible avoidance- or drug-resistant asthma while the minority may progress to end stage/dying-stage asthma. Whether it is antenatal insult or postnatal insult, there is a growing body of research data to suggest that it is the change in the pathophysiological medium of the developing lung that is paramount in the asthmagenesis process. For example, elevated anti-inflammatory cytokines have been documented during a number of antenatal events (pre-eclampsia, maternal under-nutrition) and result in a phenotype at 3 years which wheezes at the same rate as a classical group of 3-year-olds. Later in infancy, the same inflammatory marker is raised in the developing lung of children exposed to input of environmental tobacco smoke. Thus, if we stand back from the vexed argument between atopic (indoor) and non-atopic (outdoor) schools of asthma, evidence is accumulating in the form of endogenous and exogenous factors that suggest the process of early life unacceptable adverse health burden in a susceptible host has much to do with differing physiological development—neither

infectious nor allergenic—but more likely involving
immunogenic pathways and patterns of growth and repair.

2.1. Genetic Factors

It is clear that no one gene can cause the disease, but rather interactions between genetic and environmental factors are required. Moreover, the differential gene expression at specific anatomic sites is also important in contributing to the pathogenesis of childhood asthma. Therefore, combining characteristics of genetic profiles with expression patterns would be more valuable for predicting disease risk or for identifying pathways in the phenotypes of asthma. This review provides a comprehensive analysis of genetic factors in the susceptibility to and pharmacogenomic treatment of childhood asthma, focusing on genome-wide association studies (GWASs) and different candidate gene polymorphisms in major ethnic populations with childhood asthma.

There is an increasing trend in the prevalence of bronchial asthma. Genetic factors are important determinants in the pathogenesis of the disease, and heritability is typically high. Asthma is determined by the complex interplay of environmental and genetic factors. Although environmental factors have a significant role in asthma, identification of genetic predisposition is most important to get detailed insight into susceptibility of subjects to develop asthma. Currently, the major genetic types of asthma to which children tend to be affected are atopy and severe asthma. Genetic studies have identified asthma-susceptible genes in at least two pathways. Many excellent twin studies conclude that genetic factors also have a quite large contribution to the pathogenesis of childhood asthma. Thus, identifying genetic determinants of childhood asthma is particularly important in the discovery and development of specific and nontoxic targeted therapies to prevent, control, or cure this condition.

2.2. Environmental Exposures

Recognizing these environmental exposures that worsen symptoms is key as it provides grounds for interventions, including preventive measures and potentially causal treatment. Thus, exposure awareness can aid in decreasing co-morbidities and long-term end organ damage/morbidity; in primary/secondary prevention; in patient education in regards to avoidance measures and lifestyle; in supporting environmental/occupational/indoor allergy and immunotoxicology subspecialists; in avoiding misdiagnoses and unnecessary surgical intervention; and in providing potential causal treatment.

There is well-established evidence that environmental exposures contribute to both the development of asthma phenotypes and the worsening of asthma status. It is known that the vast array of pollutants in the air, water, food, and other goods that we come into contact with each day, almost innumerable, contribute to the ever-increasing prevalence of asthma amongst the pediatric population all across the globe. The wide variety of allergens that our bodies also come into contact with can worsen childhood asthma, either as the triggers for allergic responses, as is the case especially for atopic asthma, or as sources of irritants or inflammation. Some allergens that asthmatic children are exposed to include house dust mites, cockroach allergens, pet allergens, and exposure to molds sensitized individuals having mold grow in their home as a result of water intrusions. Additionally, there are a variety of other environmental triggers that can exacerbate pediatric asthma symptoms.

Huckleberry B. Hill, Kate S. Lah, Bo Morgan, Evan J. Propst, Brian K. Riff, Maria Tsoumakas, Christopher L. Carroll. Adherence of otolaryngology journals to PRISMA: 2016-2021. Laryngoscope Investigative Otolaryngology. 2022. 13(1).

2.3. Respiratory Infections

Medically, vulnerable preschool children, for example with a history of severe rhinovirus-induced wheezing and an atopic background where the mother also wets the bed after six years of age, may be selected for parent education. The goal of education is to prevent respiratory infections as much as possible. Measures could be the teaching of frequent change of bedclothes, ventilation of the room and avoidance of environmental tobacco smoke indoors. Day care attendance has been suggested to result in more frequent common colds, which could have a role in the initiation of childhood asthma. On the other hand, quality of day care might have a protective, immunostimulatory effect on asthma development as resembled to the hygiene hypothesis.

The pattern of respiratory infections shows that early (first 3 years) and recurrent respiratory infections have the strongest association with the development of recurrent wheezing or asthma, but this is also affected by the pathogenic features of the microbial agents responsible for the infections. For example, rhinovirus infections show the strongest correlation, as do the detection of more than one virus and signs of atopy. An infection in the first 3 months of life best predicts later respiratory problems and the effect is known to be strongest in families with an atopic background, especially if a severe course early in life is observed. As an anti-viral host defense, the capacity of airway epithelial cells to produce interferon has been suggested to play a preventive role. Deficient interferon production has indeed been described in cells from atopic children with asthma, an observation which matches the increased incidence of virus-induced wheezing in children of atopic patients. In viral wheezing episodes of children with and without atopic family members, responses of T cells to allergens are often observed which can last for months. Possibly the T-cells occurring in these early infections are related to the development of persistent asthma. A tentative therapeutic conclusion from these observations might be that prevention of severe virus-induced wheezing in the first years would prevent the late onset of asthma. Antivirus treatment, although an interesting concept, is still in an experimental stage. Administration of interferon in children in home settings has the limitation of local toxicity.

2.4. Exposure to Tobacco Smoke

There has been a debate over the extent to which educating parents about the hazards of passive smoking may have an effect on the rates of epidemic asthma, due to the modulating effect of the genetic predisposition on the efficacy of phenotypic or environmental information. However, as childhood asthma is epigenetically modulated, a child's lung may recover and remain free from priming after the smoking parent quits, but only if the parent quits early enough in the child's life.

Several interventions to reduce the smoking-attributable global health burden were proposed, such as legislations against smoking in public arenas, increasing tax on tobacco products, ban on marketing of tobacco products, mass-media campaigns to highlight the dangers of tobacco smoke, and access to smoking cessation programs.

Exposure to tobacco smoke at home has been associated with an increase in the risk of developing atopic sensitization, particularly if both parents smoke or have a paternal history of asthma. Regular exposure, including in utero exposure, to fumes of burnt wood, animal droppings, or other organic materials, can spike the risk of recurrent wheezing and develop early childhood asthma.

Maternal prenatal tobacco smoke exposure can upregulate the astrocytes of cytokines, such as interleukin (IL)-1 and tumor necrosis factor (TNF)-α, therefore predisposing the fetus to airway inflammation. Nicotine can cross over the placenta and be excreted in breast milk. In utero nicotine exposure was found to amplify the likelihood of children developing severe asthma with severe persistent airway obstruction.

The impact of exposure to tobacco smoke on the health of the respiratory system of children is significant. Passive smoking is a critical modifiable risk factor for pediatric asthma, mainly due to its ability to alter lung function or trigger airway remodeling. It can initiate an upsurge in the inflammatory and oxidant stress of the airways, which could last for an extended period after the cessation of exposure.

3. Diagnosis of Childhood Asthma

As a disease with complex pathogenesis and defined clinical manifestations, the diagnosis of asthma still depends on comprehensive analysis by clinicians, for which there are several diagnostic methods mentioned in the literature. A doctor will diagnose childhood asthma carried out in a few steps; the doctor will first take a medical history to follow up and explain the child's possible symptoms. It is thought to be an early symptom of asthma in children. Sometimes children with asthma do not develop typical symptoms before the wheezing and coughing occur. It may also be accompanied by allergies to food, pets, guests, pollen, and the like. A careful medical history can help your doctor make a diagnosis, can also encourage the pediatrician to do the necessary testing to ensure an accurate and timely diagnosis.

Childhood asthma is an important disease that can affect the growth and development of young children. Therefore, it is very important to diagnose the disease early and in order to get the best treatment early, many children's clinical asthma diagnostic scales and pathological diagnostic criteria can help doctors better diagnose the disease.

Childhood asthma is a common chronic disease. The current guidelines from the Global Initiative for Asthma have classified the diagnosis of asthma in children into three categories: the first is according to the clinical criteria, the second way is according to the clinical criteria and some diagnostic tests, and the third way is according to the diagnostic criteria. The purpose of diagnosing childhood asthma from the point of view of the criteria for the diagnosis of asthma is to help pediatricians better recognize, diagnose, and treat childhood asthma, so as to effectively control the condition and improve the prognosis for asthmatic children.

4. Treatment Options

Pharmacological Therapy Pharmacological therapy includes treatment that controls asthma and reduces both the severity and frequency of symptoms, as well as quick-relief medications (also known as rescue drugs or acute treatment) used to effectively treat asthma. However, medications cannot treat the underlying airway inflammation of asthma. Asthma treatment strategies proposed in the Global Initiative for Asthma guidelines are based on disease severity, treatment history, and whether prevention or rapid relief is required. After asthma is diagnosed, preferably by spirometry, classification as either intermittent or persistent helps to determine long- and short-term control options, the frequency of follow-up, and continual patient education. Intermittent asthma management requires an inhaled short-acting beta-agonist (SABA) as needed. Persistent asthma management typically requires a preferred low-dose inhaled corticosteroid (ICS) and as-needed SABA. Respecting the patients' symptoms, physical examinations, age, and preferences by setting goals is an essential component of therapy. Home environmental trigger reduction is an important step in providing comprehensive asthma care and should be incorporated into all patients' asthma action plans. Additionally, maintenance of physical conditioning when not experiencing asthma symptoms is an integral component of asthma care. Although achieving asthma control is a priority in our management objective, minimizing the need for pharmaceutical interventions is also salient. Findings in the understanding of airway inflammation in asthma sparked the development of effective, safe controller therapies. Omalizumab, Mepolizumab, clinically effective in some pediatric populations, and Dupilumab have broadened the targeted pharmacologic treatment options for children with severe asthma. While these medications are recommended for children with moderate-to-severe uncontrolled asthma, guidelines remained silent about their place in therapy for children with mild asthma, including those with a severe asthma exacerbation. Therefore, debate will continue for these cases, and the role of these medications in mild asthma remains to be defined. The search for effective and safe treatments remains an essential area of research.

Non-Pharmacological Therapy Despite a few pharmacological therapies available for asthma treatment, apart from using costly inhaled corticosteroids, the effective options to treat asthma that suppress the progression of the disease and prevent future exacerbations in children are still being explored. Thus, it is imperative to turn the focus on non-pharmacological therapies that offer prompts for children. Consequently, educating families regarding the fundamental knowledge to avoid the consequences of asthma stakeholders is crucial. Owing to the growing interest in non-pharmacological antidepressant therapy in recent years, global medical experts have explored the effectiveness of lifestyle changes. These positive activities maintain their effect on mental health and viral symptoms, which raises the need for public education on the importance of sports and lifestyle. Therefore, it seems difficult to invest because it is underestimated and sometimes obscured by wall-to-wall carpets, mattress covers, and dissolving booths.

1. Introduction 2. Etiopathogenesis of Childhood Asthma 3. Clinical Features of Childhood Asthma 4. Treatment Options 4.1. Non-Pharmacological Therapy 4.2. Pharmacological Therapy 5. Conclusions and Future Perspectives

4.1. Pharmacological Treatments

Another option for children is to use a combination inhaler of inhaled corticosteroids with a long-acting β2 adrenergic agonist for symptom management and control. Even though it is not fully understood, β2 adrenergic agonists can reduce inflammation and bradykinin-induced hyper-responsiveness in some clinical settings. In addition, there are other anti-inflammatory treatments, particularly targeted allergy desensitization treatments that can and do help treat the allergic components of the disease state, thereby reducing symptoms and risk. Biologics can be used to treat childhood asthma in moderate to severe attempts to treat with inhaled medications have failed. This review and analysis will determine pharmacological options for the treatment of childhood asthma. In understanding the pharmacological treatments of this study, providers and parents can make educated decisions and choose the best possible treatment for prevention and symptom control of asthma in children.

Pharmacological treatments: A mainstay of asthma control and symptom management in children is treating them with quick relief, short-acting β2 agonists such as albuterol, and for younger children, levalbuterol. Quick relief treatments can help unwind the bronchoconstriction and smooth muscle spasm associated with asthma exacerbations. Preventing exacerbation can be achieved with inhaled corticosteroids, systemic corticosteroids, inhaled cromones (sodium cromoglycate and nedocromil), leukotriene receptor antagonists, and long-acting β2 adrenergic agonists.

4.2. Non-Pharmacological Treatments

Clinicians have long practiced non-medical treatments to treat and manage asthma because of fears of adverse effects from drugs or because of dissatisfaction with the current medical treatments. There is evidence for the positive effects of such a complementary medical approach in the treatment of asthma in children. Yoga is said to improve ventilatory function and exercise capacity both in children and adults. Inhaling allergens, in very small doses, has been studied in children in the standardized homeopathic preparation, known as ultra-molecular agitated dilution of an allergen, also called homeopathic allergen. "Homoeopathic immunotherapy" was reported to increase peak expiratory flow rates, decrease wheeze, symptoms and reduce the use of medication in children with asthma. In the clinical approach, parents may also try naturopathies, herbal preparations, ayurvedic or traditional Chinese medicines, acupuncture and homeopathy (homeopathic remedies with an aim to balance the person's immunity across time and symptoms). Acupuncture includes the use of metal or glass needles dipped in different drugs and inserting them at specific points on the skin.

The primary strategy in the management of childhood asthma is to achieve a maximal level of control. Like other chronic diseases, reducing the impact of illness, health risks, and further psychosocial complications in children is the major aim. To maintain this, non-pharmacological management, such as regular assessment and patient education, is crucial. In addition to prescribed drugs, there are various interventions employed for non-pharmacological treatment of asthma in children. These treatments seek to help childhood asthma in a holistic way and to promote health and general well-being. They do not involve the use of drugs prescribed for ensuring good asthma control and treating acute episodes. These strategies are of importance in the entire comprehensive management of asthma in children. Non-pharmacological treatments for childhood asthma are intervention-based management strategies to avoid asthma triggers, reduce exposure to triggering factors, and prevent or manage sabotage.

5. Prevention Strategies

Screening for hereditary tolerance and early sensitization has been shown to have great value in selecting allergies or acute wheeze, so many can prevent the development of asthma in high-risk populations.

Policymakers can take steps to protect children from acquiring or exacerbating an illness. Integration between steps in various strategies, stakeholders in primary care and other healthcare settings involved in treating acute asthma symptoms, and other allergy symptoms can prevent the development of asthma.

Organizational prevention measures, including routine or as-needed surveillance of indoor and outdoor environmental incitants, outcomes such as physician diagnosing, absences from school, or health care utilization, and the effectiveness of primary prevention strategies, may use the same methods.

Practical measures may include comprehensive and individualized plans and school-based interventions, as well as checks of the effectiveness of educational intervention and environmental measures through observational or intervention trials.

Educational prevention measures include informing adults, children, and healthcare professionals about asthma prevention (e.g., the relation of environmental exposures to triggering or exacerbation, the rationale of avoiding incitants, and effective methods of limiting exposures).

Environmental measures include reducing tobacco smoke exposure, minimizing indoor allergen exposure, controlling indoor or outdoor irritants (e.g., dust mites, molds, and cockroach allergens), minimizing indoor and outdoor pollution, and minimizing harmful prenatal or postnatal environmental exposures.

Prevention of asthma is important to stem the initiation of the disease or to reduce its severity. Several strategies can be employed to prevent the onset of the disease or prevent its progress to severe disease.

Childhood asthma prevention strategies

5.1. Environmental Modifications

- Dust mite antigens can be lessened in carpeting and upholstered furnishings (e.g., sofa) by routine vacuuming with a vacuum with a small-pore bag. For a further reduction, appliances can be provided that use high-efficiency particle arresting (HEPA) or electrostatic air filters. A child with asthma probably would benefit from lessening over rugs or carpeting to zero. A child with dust mite sensitivity, or someone who might become one, would benefit most of all. Electrostatic or HEPA air cleaners, when applied in one-room, coin-opt meters at tobacco-exposed kids, were seen to give a mental health improvement concluding from the ecological, or environmental preventive, consequence of shielding these kids from inhaling tobacco smoke pollutants. Certain electrostatic or HEPA appliances can clean too little of the room volume to make a perceptible difference unless they operate in that room every day.

- Active or passive cigarette smoking in housing should be discontinued. Since smoking by visitors or the children's contact could exacerbate the child's asthma, the family may need to provide a smoke-free shelter for the child. It is necessary to assemble smoking cessation resources in the community. Under many circumstances, just a small number of smokers account for the majority of passive smoke exposures: "Ask and advise" advice for parents to quit smoking.

We should strive to make the child's living environment as "asthma friendly" as possible. Guidelines from the World Health Organization (2007) suggest simple improvements that can modify the environment to the advantage of people with asthma:

5.2. Education and Awareness Programs

School-based initiatives, supported by health professionals, to provide asthma training to both asthmatic and non-asthmatic children, and to family members, could provide a mechanism for spreading awareness about asthma management in the wider community. Studies in the UK have demonstrated that school-based interventions in which children aged 9–15 years self-managed their asthma with the support of school and community nurses achieved a reduction in hospital admissions. Furthermore, the ongoing dissemination of guidelines and education of primary healthcare providers as well as specialists about asthma is essential to maintain and improve clinical asthma control. These results provide evidence that targeted interventions in schools can improve clinical asthma control, as well as reducing asthma-related hospital services in the short-to-medium term. This highlights the potential burden of poor clinical and precautionary asthma control in children when targeted intervention in schools is absent. Interventions to educate preschool staff may also be helpful but require study in different settings.

Education and awareness programs: The development of effective education programs to improve asthma knowledge and control has received international support. Higher parental/carer knowledge of childhood asthma is associated with better asthma management. Similarly, improvements in asthma knowledge and self-efficacy in caregivers are associated with improvements in child asthma control, particularly if the child has uncontrolled symptoms at enrollment. Furthermore, parents/caregivers report that they or their children have a need for more asthma information than they have received. Overall, results from randomized trials suggest that educational interventions can improve self-management skills and reduce unscheduled healthcare utilization (hospital visits, emergency department visits) in developed countries, and have been associated with improved quality of life for children in resource-poor settings.

6. Current Research and Innovations

These studies demonstrate advances in our understanding of the etiological phases of asthma including molecular and cellular endotypes, the role of lung immune and structural cells in the pathogenesis of asthma, and the epidemiology and relationships between lifestyle factors for asthma. The customized and integrated management principles require further development, including the role of bi-responsive and T2 therapies, the role of macrophages and many novel treatments, vaccine studies and modifications of the environment.

Asthma management in pediatric age – urgency of development of a chronic care model.

Vaida Siupsinskaite, Veslav Kopriva, Vaida Kvedaraite Sarzuet, Birute Strakonien and Rasa Jasinskaja-La

High-intensity interval training in asthma: From mechanisms to clinical practice.

Kanjutra VanThu, Richard J. Martin and Yi Zheng

Intravital microscopy imaging of platelet-leukocyte interactions and MMP12 expressing plasmacytoid dendritic cells associated with airway inflammation in asthma.

Jiawei Zhou, Nga Chun, Anthony Lin-Brande, Lotus Francis, Jeongni Lee, Rebecca Heavy, Jonathan Tomaszewski, Imran

Khan, Cyrus N. Manuel, Serhan Inceoglu and Jessica Wagoner

Fatty Acids and Exosomal miRNAs for Metabolic Dysregulation in Childhood Asthma.

Kairui Mao, Guicheng Chen, Ying Cao and Cui Qu

Methionine restriction in early-life with a high-fat diet hampers the early-life asthmatic immune milieu in offspring despite post-weaning correction.

Layla Ballang, Tamara Jones, Karlie McLaughlan, Joseph M. Collaco, Rita Stoppa and Philip J. Thompson

7. Conclusion and Future Directions

In summary, we have discussed that at the time of the final diagnosis of childhood asthma aggression, it is common for dust mite sensitivity, IgE, AD, inhaled corticosteroids, viral triggers, and clinical diagnostic history very high. These critical drives might be targeted several years earlier than the study described in this review and have significant future potential as a combined disease-modifying therapy aimed at slowing or reversing the progression of asthma at a time when the disease is still potentially preventable - with a holding bonus. The data confirming that antigen avoidance or immunotherapy might have disease-remodifying benefits have largely been focusing on relatively small studies conducted among children with relatively mild to moderate asthma and combined with adults. To our knowledge, no prior childhood asthma prevention study conducted affected older children at a later asthma point eligible. While recruitment to the study proposed here is undoubtedly possible, potential subjects might require much more frequent clinic visits in the early part of the groin and weekly aerosol challenges to ensure compliance with the dosing regime.

In addition, the likelihood of a consistent airway abnormality or deficit as the direct cause of immune activity is extremely low early in the childhood asthma process, as shown by the many different immune and inflammatory "causes" associated with childhood asthma diagnosis. An injectable, targeted IL-4 antagonist, dupilumab, significantly improved lung function and reduced exacerbations in children with uncontrolled moderate-to-severe asthma, satisfying the primary endpoint and showing a consistent and comprehensive atopic and nonatopic steroid-sparing benefit. Anti-TSLP monoclonal antibodies and house dust mite sublingual immunotherapy have shown clinically meaningful improvements in asthma control, accompanied by some evidence of a steroid-sparing effect. Several novel therapeutics isolated through overlapping pathways are now being tested in children at an early stage in their asthma trajectory, prior to lung function deterioration, in the hope that the trial and validation needed to prove disease efficacy and successful disease-modification thriller signals in key clinical trials can be achieved. Amazingly, recent studies have demonstrated that the very first cause of childhood asthma effectively preventable with omalizumab at 18-24 months is effectively preventable, providing hope for future primary prevention studies using these methods.

Many asthma studies find that the relationships between identified "causes" from observational studies and the initiation of childhood asthma are merely plausibly associated with disease activity and are discovered indirectly by using cross-sectional associations between detected susceptible phenotypes and current asthma activity (i.e., reverse causation).

Childhood asthma continues to be a major issue for public health, with a variety of underlying causes. Although numerous factors contributing to asthma have been demonstrated in humans and animal models, their relative importance and potential interactions are still largely unknown. This review is based on our current understanding of the causes of asthma and sets out its significance for the understanding of the initiation process, subsequent progression, and potential new avenues of treatment.